The Plant-Powered Living

Transform Your Health, Reverse, and Prevent Chronic Diseases with a Whole Food Plant-Based Diet

Dr. Myles Watson Collins

About the Author

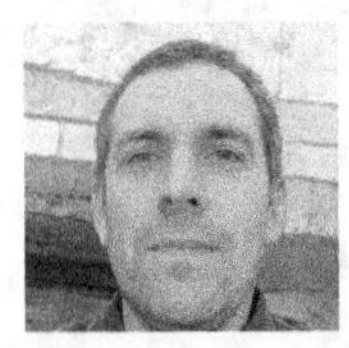 Dr. Myles Watson Collins is a leading nutritionist and health expert with over 20 years of experience in the field. He holds a Ph.D. in Nutrition from Harvard University and is a certified dietitian. Dr. Collins has dedicated his career to studying the impact of diet on health and disease prevention.

In addition to his work at the hospital, Dr. Collins also runs the Revitalize Wellness Center, a premier wellness facility located in the heart of New York City, where he offers personalized nutrition and wellness plans, fitness programs, and stress management to help individuals achieve optimal health through natural and science-backed methods.

Dr. Collins is also a certified Plant-Based Health Coach. He anchors the Plant Powered Life program, where he coaches individuals to make plant-based eating simple, easy, and delicious. Dr. Collins and his dedicated team work tirelessly to help individuals achieve their health goals and improve their quality of life.

Dr. Collins is an avid writer and has contributed numerous articles to prestigious newspapers and journals, including *The New York Times*, *The Washington Post*, *Health Journal*, and *Nutrition Science Review*. His research focuses on the benefits of whole foods, the role of macronutrients and micronutrients in health, and the prevention of chronic diseases through diet.

In addition to his research, Dr. Collins has worked with various health organizations to develop nutrition guidelines and educational materials. He is passionate about making nutrition information accessible and practical for everyone.

Dr. Collins's dedication to improving public health through nutrition education has earned him numerous awards and recognition. He continues to inspire and educate others on the importance of healthy eating and lifestyle choices.

In addition to his professional accomplishments, Dr. Collins is an avid cyclist and enjoys exploring the scenic routes of New York. He is also a passionate cook, often experimenting with new healthy recipes that he shares with his clients and followers. He enjoys gardening, which he finds to be a relaxing and rewarding hobby as well. He believes that growing his own vegetables not only supports his family's health but also deepens his connection with nature.

Dr. Collins lives in Brooklyn, New York, with his wife, Kathleen, and their three children, Rebecca, Deborah, and James. His family is his greatest source of inspiration and support. Dr. Collins' commitment to his family and his community is reflected in his dedication to promoting healthy living and wellness for all.

Dr. Collins's passion for Optimal health extends beyond his professional and writing endeavors. He frequently speaks at conferences and seminars, sharing his knowledge and inspiring others to take charge of their health through better nutrition, diet, and lifestyle choices.

Dear Readers,

If you enjoyed reading and using this book, please leave a review. Your feedback means a lot to me and helps others discover the book. I will really appreciate it.

Thank you!

Contents

Introduction

Jenny had tried everything—fad diets, calorie counting, grueling exercise routines—yet nothing seemed to work. In her early 40s, she found herself battling with stubborn weight gain, creeping blood pressure, and fatigue that never seemed to lift. Every visit to the doctor left her with more prescriptions and fewer answers. Deep down, she feared that her future would mirror her parents', who had struggled with heart disease and diabetes, believing it was just a matter of genetics.

But everything changed when Jenny stumbled upon the idea of a whole food plant-based diet. Skeptical at first, she decided to give it a try, not expecting much. Within weeks, she noticed a shift—not just in her weight, but in her energy, her mood, and most importantly, her health markers. Her blood pressure normalized, her cholesterol dropped, and for the first time in years, she felt truly alive. Jenny had discovered a secret that would not only transform her health but change her life forever.

Welcome to "The Plant-Powered Living: Transform Your Health, Reverse and Prevent Chronic Diseases with a Whole Food Plant-Based Diet." This book is your guide to discovering the incredible power of plants to heal, nourish, and energize your body. Like Jenny, you may have been led to believe that chronic diseases, weight gain, and declining energy are inevitable parts of aging. But what if that's not the case? What if you could take control of your health, defy your genetic predispositions, and live a vibrant, energized life?

The primary goal of this book is to show you that it's possible. Through the pages of this book, you'll learn how a whole food plant-based diet can be your roadmap to health transformation. This isn't just another diet fad or temporary fix. This is about adopting a lifestyle that aligns with the natural rhythms of your body, allowing it to function at its best.

What You Will Learn:

The Truth About Chronic Diseases: Understand how many chronic diseases are not just genetic fates but can be prevented and even reversed through lifestyle changes.

The Science of Plant-Based Nutrition: Discover the research-backed benefits of a whole food plant-based diet, including its power to reduce inflammation, improve heart health, and boost energy levels.

Practical Steps to Transition: Learn how to gradually shift to a plant-based lifestyle with easy-to-follow tips on meal planning, grocery shopping, and nutrition essentials.

Delicious Recipes: Enjoy a variety of tasty and satisfying plant-based recipes for every meal of the day, from breakfast to dinner, snacks, and even drinks.

Real-Life Success Stories: Be inspired by the journeys of people like Jenny who have transformed their health and lives through the power of plants.

This book is more than just a guide—it's an invitation to reclaim your health, renew your energy, and rediscover the joy of eating whole, natural foods. Whether you're looking to lose weight, boost your energy, or prevent disease, this book provides the roadmap to take control of your health destiny.

Don't settle for mediocrity—take the first step toward a healthier, happier you. Embrace the plant-powered life today and watch your health soar!

Chapter 1: The Myth of Genetic Predestination

Understanding Genetic Myths

Many people believe that if their parents or grandparents had chronic diseases like heart disease, diabetes, or cancer, they are destined to have these diseases too. This belief is based on the idea that our genes control our health completely, leaving us with no power to change our health outcomes. This chapter will show you why this belief is not true and how you can take control of your health.

Common Misconceptions About Genetics and Chronic Diseases

1. **Genetics as Destiny**: One of the biggest misconceptions is that if a disease runs in your family, you will definitely get it. While genes do play a role, they are not the only factor.

2. **Unchangeable Health**: Many people think that their health is fixed and unchangeable because of their genes. This belief makes them feel powerless and less motivated to make healthy choices.

3. **Ignoring Lifestyle**: Some believe that since genes determine health, lifestyle choices like diet and exercise do not matter. This leads to neglecting important habits that can improve health.

4. **The Role of Genetics vs. Lifestyle Choices**

It's important to understand that genes do influence our health, but they are not the sole factor. In fact, lifestyle choices have a significant impact on whether or not we develop chronic diseases. Here's how:

Genes Load the Gun, Lifestyle Pulls the Trigger

This saying means that while genes may create a potential for disease, lifestyle choices determine whether that potential is realized. For example, someone may have a genetic predisposition to diabetes, but if they eat a healthy diet and exercise regularly, they may never develop the disease.

Epigenetics: How Lifestyle Changes Genes

Epigenetics is the study of how our behaviors and environment can cause changes that affect the way our genes work. Unlike genetic changes, epigenetic changes are reversible and do not change your DNA sequence, but they can change how your body reads a DNA sequence. For instance, a plant-based diet can switch on genes that protect against diseases and switch off genes that promote disease.

The Role of Diet

What we eat plays a crucial role in determining our health. A diet high in fruits, vegetables, whole grains, and legumes can protect against chronic diseases, even if you have a genetic predisposition. Conversely, a diet high in processed foods, sugar, and unhealthy fats can increase the risk of these diseases.

The Role of Exercise

Regular physical activity can also influence how our genes are expressed. Exercise can reduce the risk of heart disease, diabetes, and other chronic conditions by improving metabolism, reducing inflammation, and promoting healthy blood flow.

Stress Management and Sleep

Managing stress and getting enough sleep are also important. Chronic stress and poor sleep can negatively impact gene expression, leading to increased risk of chronic diseases. Practices like meditation, yoga, and good sleep hygiene can positively affect our health.

The Impact of Lifestyle

How Lifestyle Changes Can Influence Health

When you adopt a healthy lifestyle, you can significantly reduce your risk of chronic diseases, even if you have a genetic predisposition. Here's how lifestyle changes can make a difference:

Improving Diet

Switching to a whole food plant-based diet can provide your body with the nutrients it needs to function properly. This type of diet is rich in fiber, vitamins, minerals, and antioxidants, which can help prevent and even reverse chronic diseases.

Increasing Physical Activity

Incorporating regular exercise into your routine can strengthen your heart, improve your metabolism, and boost your immune system. Even simple activities like walking, gardening, or dancing can make a big difference.

Managing Stress

Learning to manage stress through techniques like meditation, deep breathing, or spending time in nature can reduce inflammation and improve overall health. Chronic stress can lead to a variety of health issues, so finding ways to relax and unwind is crucial.

Getting Enough Sleep

Quality sleep is essential for maintaining health. Poor sleep can lead to weight gain, diabetes, and heart disease. Establishing a regular sleep schedule and creating a restful environment can help improve sleep quality.

Real-World Examples and Studies

Study on Heart Disease

A landmark study by Dr. Dean Ornish showed that a whole food plant-based diet, combined with regular exercise, stress management, and social support, can not only prevent but also reverse heart disease. Patients who followed this lifestyle saw significant improvements in their heart health, regardless of their genetic predisposition.

Study on Diabetes

Research by Dr. Neal Barnard demonstrated that a low-fat plant-based diet can improve insulin sensitivity and reduce blood sugar levels in people with type 2 diabetes. Many participants were able to reduce or eliminate their need for medication.

Study on Cancer

Studies have shown that a plant-based diet can reduce the risk of certain types of cancer. For example, populations that consume a diet rich in fruits, vegetables, and whole grains have lower rates of colon, breast, and prostate cancer.

Lessons Learned

1. **Genes are not Destiny**: Your health is not solely determined by your genes. Lifestyle choices play a significant role in your overall health.
2. **You Have the Power**: By making healthy choices, you can take control of your health destiny. This includes adopting a plant-based diet, exercising regularly, managing stress, and getting enough sleep.
3. **Start Small**: Even small changes can have a big impact. Begin by incorporating more fruits and vegetables into your diet, taking short walks, and finding ways to relax.
4. **Be Consistent**: Consistency is key. Making healthy choices a regular part of your routine will lead to lasting improvements in your health.

5. **Seek Support**: Surround yourself with supportive people who encourage your healthy lifestyle. Join a community, find a buddy, or seek guidance from a health coach.

The belief that chronic diseases are inevitable and unchangeable is a myth. While genetics do play a role, lifestyle choices have a significant impact on your health. By adopting a whole food plant-based diet, exercising regularly, managing stress, and getting enough sleep, you can take control of your health destiny. This chapter has shown that you have the power to make a difference in your health, regardless of your genetic predisposition. The following chapters will provide more detailed guidance on how to implement these changes and transform your life.

Chapter 2: The Science Behind Plant-Based Nutrition

What is a Whole Food Plant-Based Diet?

Definition and Core Principles

A whole food plant-based (WFPB) diet focuses on consuming natural, minimally processed plant foods. It emphasizes the intake of fruits, vegetables, whole grains, legumes, nuts, and seeds. The core principles of a WFPB diet include:

- **Whole Foods**: Foods that are in their natural state, with minimal processing and no added chemicals or prescrvatives. This means eating fruits, vegetables, whole grains, and legumes as they are found in nature.
- **Plant-Based**: Avoiding animal products like meat, dairy, and eggs. Instead, focusing on plant-derived foods for all nutritional needs.

- **Minimally Processed**: Choosing foods that are as close to their natural form as possible. This means avoiding refined sugars, oils, and processed foods.
- **Rich in Nutrients**: A WFPB diet is packed with vitamins, minerals, fiber, and antioxidants that are essential for maintaining good health.
- **Low in Unhealthy Fats**: This diet limits the intake of unhealthy fats found in animal products and processed foods, emphasizing healthy fats from plant sources like avocados, nuts, and seeds.

Health Benefits

Overview of Health Benefits Supported by Scientific Research

A WFPB diet offers numerous health benefits, which are supported by a growing body of scientific research. These benefits include:

- **Reduced Risk of Chronic Diseases**: Studies have shown that a plant-based diet can lower the risk of heart disease, diabetes, cancer, and other chronic conditions.
- **Improved Heart Health**: Consuming a diet rich in fruits, vegetables, whole grains, and legumes can help reduce cholesterol levels, lower blood pressure, and improve overall heart health.
- **Better Weight Management**: A WFPB diet is naturally lower in calories and high in fiber, which can help with weight loss and maintaining a healthy weight.
- **Enhanced Digestive Health**: The high fiber content in plant foods promotes healthy digestion and prevents constipation.
- **Increased Energy Levels**: Plant-based foods provide essential nutrients that can boost energy levels and improve overall vitality.

- **Improved Mental Health**: Research suggests that a plant-based diet can positively impact mental health, reducing symptoms of depression and anxiety.

Key Studies and Findings

1. **The China Study**: This comprehensive study by Dr. T. Colin Campbell and Dr. Thomas M. Campbell II examined the relationship between diet and disease in rural China. The findings showed that diets high in animal protein were linked to higher rates of chronic diseases, while plant-based diets were associated with lower rates of these diseases.

2. **The Adventist Health Studies**: These studies conducted on Seventh-day Adventists, who often follow a plant-based diet, found that plant-based eaters had lower rates of heart disease, diabetes, and certain cancers compared to the general population.

3. **Dr. Dean Ornish's Studies**: Dr. Ornish's research demonstrated that a low-fat plant-based diet, combined with lifestyle changes, could reverse heart disease. Patients showed significant improvements in their heart health, including reduced arterial blockages.

4. **The EPIC-Oxford Study**: This large-scale study found that vegetarians and vegans had lower risks of heart disease and cancer compared to meat-eaters. It also highlighted the importance of plant-based nutrition in overall health.

5. **Dr. Caldwell Esselstyn's Research**: Dr. Esselstyn's work at the Cleveland Clinic showed that a whole food plant-based diet could halt and even reverse advanced heart disease. His patients experienced significant improvements in their heart health and quality of life.

Preventing and Reversing Diseases

**How Plant-Based Nutrition Addresses the
Root Cause of Chronic Diseases**

A WFPB diet addresses the root cause of chronic diseases by reducing inflammation, improving blood flow, and promoting overall health. Here's how it works:

- **Reduces Inflammation**: Plant-based foods are rich in antioxidants and phytonutrients that help reduce inflammation, a key factor in many chronic diseases.
- **Improves Blood Flow**: A diet low in unhealthy fats and high in fiber helps improve blood flow and reduces the risk of arterial blockages.
- **Promotes Healthy Weight**: Maintaining a healthy weight through a plant-based diet reduces the risk of many chronic diseases, including heart disease, diabetes, and certain cancers.

- **Lowers Cholesterol Levels**: A WFPB diet naturally lowers cholesterol levels, reducing the risk of heart disease and stroke.
- **Regulates Blood Sugar**: Plant-based foods, especially whole grains and legumes, help regulate blood sugar levels, reducing the risk of type 2 diabetes.

Case Studies and Expert Opinions

Case Study 1: John's Heart Disease Reversal

John, a 52-year-old man with a history of heart disease, was able to reverse his condition by switching to a WFPB diet. After just six months, his cholesterol levels dropped significantly, and his arterial blockages were reduced. John's case is a testament to the power of plant-based nutrition in reversing heart disease.

Case Study 2: Flora's Diabetes Management

Flora, a 45-year-old woman diagnosed with type 2 diabetes, managed to control her blood sugar levels and reduce her medication by adopting a plant-based diet. Within a year, Flora's HbA1c levels returned to normal, and she felt more energetic and healthier than ever before.

The importance of a WFPB diet in preventing and reversing chronic diseases cannot be overemphasized. It is observed that the best way to fight chronic diseases is to prevent them in the first place with a healthy diet. And if you're already suffering from a chronic condition, a plant-based diet can help you reverse it.

It is also noted that a plant-based diet is a powerful tool for preventing and reversing many of the leading causes of death and disability. The science is clear: plant-based diets are good for your health.

It is also noted that heart disease need not exist, and if it does exist, it need not progress. The key to this transformation is a whole food plant-based diet.

The science behind plant-based nutrition is robust and compelling. A whole food plant-based diet not only provides essential nutrients but also plays a crucial role in preventing and reversing chronic diseases. The health benefits are supported by numerous studies and expert opinions, demonstrating that a plant-based lifestyle can significantly improve overall health and well-being.

In the next chapter, we will delve into the practical aspects of following a plant-based diet, including how to meet your nutritional needs and debunking common myths. By understanding the science and applying it to your daily life, you can take control of your health and enjoy the many benefits of plant-based nutrition.

Chapter 3: Nutrition Essentials on a Plant-Based Diet

Meeting Nutritional Needs

When adopting a plant-based diet, it's important to ensure that you get all the necessary nutrients your body needs to function optimally. Here's how to meet your nutritional needs for protein, calcium, vitamin B12, vitamin D, omega-3s, and more.

Protein

Many people worry about getting enough protein on a plant-based diet. However, there are plenty of plant-based sources of protein that can meet your needs.

- **Legumes**: Beans, lentils, chickpeas, and peas are excellent sources of protein.

- **Nuts and Seeds**: Almonds, walnuts, chia seeds, flaxseeds, and sunflower seeds provide protein and healthy fats.
- **Whole Grains**: Quinoa, brown rice, oats, and barley are good protein sources.
- **Vegetables**: Spinach, broccoli, and Brussels sprouts contain protein.
- **Soy Products**: Tofu, tempeh, and edamame are high in protein.

To ensure you get enough protein, aim to include a variety of these foods in your meals throughout the day.

Calcium

Calcium is essential for bone health, and there are plenty of plant-based sources of calcium.

- **Leafy Greens**: Kale, collard greens, and bok choy are rich in calcium.
- **Fortified Plant Milks**: Almond milk, soy milk, and rice milk are often fortified with calcium.

- **Tofu**: Some tofu is made with calcium sulfate, which boosts its calcium content.
- **Almonds**: A good source of calcium and healthy fats.
- **Sesame Seeds and Tahini**: High in calcium.

Include these foods regularly to ensure adequate calcium intake.

Vitamin B12

Vitamin B12 is crucial for nerve function and the production of DNA and red blood cells. Since B12 is primarily found in animal products, those on a plant-based diet need to find alternative sources.

- **Fortified Foods**: Nutritional yeast, fortified plant milks, and fortified cereals.
- **Supplements**: Taking a B12 supplement can ensure you meet your needs.

Vitamin D

Vitamin D is important for bone health and immune function. While the body can produce vitamin D through sunlight exposure, dietary sources are also important.

- **Sunlight**: Spend time outdoors in the sun to help your body produce vitamin D.
- **Fortified Foods**: Fortified plant milks and cereals.
- **Mushrooms**: Some mushrooms exposed to UV light are good sources of vitamin D.
- **Supplements**: A vitamin D supplement can help, especially in winter or for those with limited sun exposure.

Omega-3 Fatty Acids

Omega-3s are essential for heart and brain health. While they are abundant in fish, plant-based sources are also available.

- **Flaxseeds**: Ground flaxseeds can be added to smoothies, oatmeal, or baked goods.
- **Chia Seeds**: High in omega-3s and can be added to many dishes.
- **Walnuts**: A great source of omega-3s and other nutrients.
- **Hemp Seeds**: Can be sprinkled on salads, cereals, or added to smoothies.
- **Algal Oil**: Derived from algae, this supplement provides DHA and EPA, the most beneficial forms of omega-3s.

Debunking Myths

Myth: Plant-Based Diets Lack Protein

As mentioned earlier, plant-based diets can provide ample protein through a variety of sources. Combining different protein-rich foods throughout the day ensures you meet your protein needs.

Myth: You Can't Get Enough Calcium Without Dairy

Many plant-based foods are rich in calcium, and fortified plant milks provide as much calcium as dairy milk. By including a variety of these foods, you can easily meet your calcium requirements.

Myth: Vitamin B12 Deficiency is Inevitable

While B12 is not naturally abundant in plant foods, fortified foods and supplements can provide adequate amounts. Regular intake of these sources can prevent deficiency.

Myth: Plant-Based Diets are Always Low in Iron

Iron is available in plant foods such as lentils, chickpeas, beans, and fortified cereals. Consuming vitamin C-rich foods (like citrus fruits, tomatoes, and bell peppers) with iron-rich meals can enhance iron absorption.

Myth: Plant-Based Diets are Expensive

Whole plant foods like beans, rice, and seasonal vegetables are often less expensive than meat and dairy products. Planning meals and buying in bulk can help keep costs down.

Balanced Eating

Tips for Creating Balanced, Nutrient-Rich Meals

Creating balanced meals on a plant-based diet is straightforward and enjoyable. Here are some tips:

- **Variety**: Include a wide range of fruits, vegetables, whole grains, legumes, nuts, and seeds in your diet to ensure you get a broad spectrum of nutrients.
- **Colorful Plates**: Aim to have a variety of colors on your plate. Different colors in fruits and vegetables indicate different nutrients.

- **Whole Foods**: Focus on whole, unprocessed foods to get the maximum nutritional benefit.
- **Protein with Every Meal**: Include a source of protein with each meal, such as beans, lentils, tofu, or nuts.
- **Healthy Fats**: Add healthy fats like avocados, nuts, seeds, and olive oil to your meals.
- **Hydration**: Drink plenty of water throughout the day to stay hydrated.
- **Meal Planning**: Plan your meals and snacks ahead of time to ensure you have balanced options available.

Supplementation

When and How to Use Supplements

While a well-planned plant-based diet can provide most of the nutrients you need, some people may benefit from supplements to ensure they meet their nutritional needs. Here's when and how to use supplements:

Vitamin B12: As mentioned, B12 is essential and should be taken as a supplement or consumed through fortified foods regularly.

Vitamin D: If you don't get enough sunlight or consume fortified foods, consider taking a vitamin D supplement, especially during the winter months.

Omega-3s: If you don't consume enough flaxseeds, chia seeds, or walnuts, consider taking an algal oil supplement to ensure adequate DHA and EPA intake.

Iron: If you are at risk of iron deficiency or have low iron levels, an iron supplement may be necessary. Consult with a healthcare provider for appropriate dosing.

Calcium: While it's possible to get enough calcium from plant foods, those who don't may benefit from a calcium supplement.

Multivitamin: A good quality multivitamin can cover any potential gaps in your diet, especially during the transition to a plant-based lifestyle.

Meeting your nutritional needs on a plant-based diet is entirely possible with careful planning and consideration. By focusing on a variety of whole, minimally processed plant foods, you can ensure that you get enough protein, calcium, vitamin B12, vitamin D, omega-3s, and other essential nutrients. Debunking common myths about plant-based diets can help you make informed choices and maintain a balanced, nutrient-rich diet. Supplementation, when necessary, can provide additional support to ensure you meet your nutritional requirements.

In the next chapter, we will explore how a plant-based diet can help with weight loss without deprivation, offering practical tips and strategies for successful weight management.

Chapter 4: Weight Loss Without Deprivation

The Plant-Based Advantage

Switching to a plant-based diet is one of the most effective ways to lose weight without feeling deprived. Unlike many fad diets that emphasize restriction and calorie counting, a whole food plant-based diet allows you to eat satisfying, nutrient-dense foods that naturally promote weight loss. Here's how a plant-based diet aids weight loss:

Low-Calorie Density

Plant-based foods are typically lower in calories but higher in volume compared to animal products and processed foods. This means you can eat larger portions, feel full, and still consume fewer calories. Foods like vegetables, fruits, whole grains, and legumes are rich in water and fiber, contributing to their low-calorie density.

High Fiber Content

Fiber is a key component of plant-based foods that aids in weight loss. It helps you feel full longer, reduces cravings, and stabilizes blood sugar levels. High-fiber foods include fruits, vegetables, whole grains, and legumes. Fiber also promotes healthy digestion and regular bowel movements, which are essential for weight management.

Nutrient-Rich Foods

A whole food plant-based diet is packed with essential nutrients that support overall health and weight loss. Vitamins, minerals, antioxidants, and phytochemicals found in plant foods help boost metabolism, reduce inflammation, and promote fat loss. Nutrient-dense foods provide your body with the necessary fuel to function optimally while reducing the risk of overeating.

Balanced Blood Sugar Levels

Plant-based diets, particularly those rich in whole grains and legumes, help maintain stable blood sugar levels. Stable blood sugar levels prevent insulin spikes and crashes, reducing the likelihood of storing excess fat. This balance also reduces cravings and helps control appetite.

Eating More, Weighing Less

One of the most appealing aspects of a plant-based diet is the ability to eat more food while still losing weight. This approach contrasts sharply with traditional dieting, which often involves strict portion control and calorie restriction. Here are some strategies for feeling full and satisfied on a plant-based diet:

Focus on Whole Foods

Whole foods are unprocessed and retain their natural fiber, which helps you feel full. Examples include fresh fruits, vegetables, whole grains, beans, and legumes. These foods provide bulk without excessive calories.

Include Protein-Rich Plants

Plant-based protein sources like beans, lentils, tofu, tempeh, and quinoa are satisfying and help maintain muscle mass during weight loss. Including a source of plant protein with every meal can keep you full and energized.

Eat Plenty of Vegetables

Vegetables are low in calories but high in volume and nutrients. Incorporate a variety of colorful vegetables into your meals to increase satiety and add essential vitamins and minerals.

Don't Skip Healthy Fats

Healthy fats from avocados, nuts, seeds, and olive oil can help you feel full and satisfied. These fats are important for brain health, hormone production, and overall well-being.

Include small amounts of healthy fats in your meals to enhance flavor and satiety.

Drink Water

Staying hydrated is crucial for weight loss and overall health. Sometimes thirst is mistaken for hunger, leading to unnecessary snacking. Drink water throughout the day, and consider having a glass of water before meals to aid digestion and help control appetite.

Practical Tips

Achieving and maintaining a healthy weight on a plant-based diet is entirely feasible with the right approach. Here are some practical tips for successful weight management:

Plan Your Meals

Meal planning helps you stay on track and make healthier choices. Plan your meals and snacks for the week, focusing on whole, plant-based foods. Preparing meals in advance can prevent impulsive eating and reliance on convenience foods.

Read Labels

When purchasing packaged foods, read labels carefully to avoid hidden sugars, unhealthy fats, and excessive sodium. Opt for products with minimal ingredients and no artificial additives.

Avoid Processed Foods

Even on a plant-based diet, processed foods like vegan junk food can hinder weight loss. These foods are often high in calories, sugar, and unhealthy fats. Stick to whole, unprocessed foods as much as possible.

Practice Mindful Eating

Pay attention to your hunger and fullness cues. Eat slowly and savor each bite. Avoid distractions like TV or smartphones while eating, as they can lead to overeating.

Stay Active

Regular physical activity is essential for weight loss and overall health. Find activities you enjoy, such as walking, cycling, swimming, or yoga, and incorporate them into your routine. Aim for at least 150 minutes of moderate-intensity exercise per week.

Get Enough Sleep

Sleep is crucial for weight management. Lack of sleep can disrupt hormones that regulate hunger and appetite, leading to weight gain. Aim for 7-9 hours of quality sleep per night.

Overcoming Challenges

Transitioning to a plant-based diet and maintaining weight loss can come with challenges. Here are some common obstacles and strategies to overcome them:

Cravings for Unhealthy Foods

Cravings for unhealthy foods can be challenging, especially when transitioning to a plant-based diet. Combat cravings by ensuring your meals are satisfying and balanced. Keep healthy snacks on hand, such as fruits, nuts, or hummus with vegetables. If cravings persist, allow yourself occasional treats in moderation to avoid feelings of deprivation.

Social Situations and Eating Out

Social events and dining out can be difficult when following a plant-based diet. Plan ahead by researching restaurant menus and choosing places with plant-based options. Don't hesitate to ask for modifications to make dishes plant-based. Bring a plant-based dish to social gatherings to ensure there's something you can eat.

Limited Access to Plant-Based Foods

If you live in an area with limited access to plant-based foods, focus on staples like beans, lentils, rice, oats, and frozen vegetables, which are often available and affordable. Consider growing your own vegetables if you have the space and resources.

Nutritional Deficiencies

Ensuring you get all necessary nutrients on a plant-based diet can be challenging. Regularly include a variety of nutrient-dense foods in your diet and consider supplements for nutrients like vitamin B12, vitamin D, and omega-3s if needed.

Time Constraints

Preparing plant-based meals can seem time-consuming, but with some planning, it can be manageable. Batch cooking, using a slow cooker, and preparing simple meals can save time. Keep quick and easy options like canned beans, frozen vegetables, and whole grains on hand for busy days.

A whole food plant-based diet offers a sustainable and enjoyable way to achieve and maintain a healthy weight without feeling deprived. By focusing on nutrient-dense foods, practicing mindful eating, and staying active, you can successfully manage your weight and improve your overall health. While challenges may arise, practical strategies and a positive mindset can help you overcome them and stay on track. In the next chapter, we will explore a simple roadmap to transition to a plant-based lifestyle, including meal planning, grocery shopping, and maintaining the lifestyle long-term.

Chapter 5: A Simple Roadmap to Transitioning to a Whole Food Plant-Based Lifestyle

Step-by-Step Guide

Transitioning to a whole food plant-based lifestyle can seem daunting at first, but with a clear roadmap, it becomes much more manageable. Here are practical steps to help you make the transition smoothly and sustainably.

Start Slow

- **Assess Your Current Diet**: Take note of what you currently eat and identify areas where you can incorporate more plant-based foods.
- **Begin with One Meal**: Start by making one meal a day completely plant-based. Breakfast is often the easiest to change—try oatmeal with

fruits and nuts or a smoothie packed with greens and berries.

- **Gradually Increase Plant-Based Meals**: Once you're comfortable with one plant-based meal a day, gradually increase to two meals, and then three. This slow transition helps your body and taste buds adjust.

Educate Yourself

- **Read Books and Articles**: Educate yourself about the benefits of a plant-based diet. The more you know, the more motivated you'll be.
- **Watch Documentaries**: Films like "Forks Over Knives" and "What the Health" provide compelling information about plant-based nutrition.
- **Join Online Communities**: Connect with others who are on the same journey. Online forums and social media groups can offer support, recipes, and tips.

Experiment with New Recipes

- **Try New Foods**: Explore different plant-based foods and recipes. Experimenting with new ingredients and cooking methods can make the transition exciting.
- **Keep it Simple**: Start with simple recipes that require minimal ingredients and time. As you get more comfortable, you can try more complex dishes.

Meal Planning and Preparation

Meal planning and preparation are key to successfully transitioning to a plant-based diet. Here are some tips to help you get started:

Plan Your Meals

- **Weekly Planning**: Dedicate some time each week to plan your meals. Write down what you'll eat for breakfast, lunch, dinner, and snacks. This helps you stay organized and ensures you have all the ingredients you need.

- **Balanced Meals**: Ensure your meals include a balance of vegetables, fruits, whole grains, legumes, nuts, and seeds. This variety will help you get all the necessary nutrients.

Batch Cooking

- **Cook in Batches**: Prepare large quantities of staples like beans, grains, and roasted vegetables that can be used throughout the week. Store them in the refrigerator or freezer for easy access.
- **Pre-Cut Vegetables**: Cut vegetables in advance and store them in the fridge. This saves time during the week and makes it easier to throw together quick meals.

Simple Recipes

- **Go-To Meals**: Have a few go-to recipes that you can make quickly. Examples include stir-fries, salads, soups, and grain bowls.
- **One-Pot Meals**: One-pot meals like stews and casseroles are convenient and minimize cleanup.

Grocery Shopping

Knowing how to shop for whole food plant-based ingredients is essential. Here are some tips to make your grocery shopping efficient and effective:

Make a List

- **Plan Ahead**: Based on your meal plan, make a shopping list of all the ingredients you need. Stick to the list to avoid impulse buys.
- **Categorize Items**: Organize your list by categories (e.g., produce, grains, legumes) to make shopping quicker and more efficient.

Shop the Perimeter

- **Focus on Fresh Foods**: The perimeter of the grocery store typically contains fresh produce, whole grains, and other whole foods. Spend most of your time here.
- **Avoid Processed Foods**: Try to avoid the inner aisles that often contain processed and packaged foods.

Buy in Bulk

- **Bulk Bins**: Many stores have bulk sections where you can buy grains, beans, nuts, and seeds. This can save money and reduce packaging waste.
- **Stock Up**: Buy larger quantities of staple items when they are on sale.

Seasonal and Local Produce

- **Buy Seasonal**: Seasonal produce is often fresher and more affordable. Look for what's in season in your area.

- **Support Local Farmers**: Shopping at farmers' markets can provide access to fresh, locally-grown produce.

Read Labels

- **Check Ingredients**: When buying packaged foods, read the ingredient list. Aim for products with minimal, recognizable ingredients and avoid added sugars, oils, and preservatives.

Maintaining the Lifestyle

Making sustainable changes is key to maintaining a plant-based lifestyle long-term. Here are strategies to help you stick with it:

Find Support

- **Connect with Others**: Join plant-based groups or communities, either locally or online. Sharing your journey with others can provide motivation and support.

- **Family Involvement**: If possible, involve your family in your new eating habits. Cooking and eating together can make the transition easier and more enjoyable.

Stay Informed

- **Keep Learning**: Continue to educate yourself about plant-based nutrition and health benefits. Staying informed can help you stay motivated.
- **Stay Updated**: Follow plant-based blogs, podcasts, and social media accounts to get new recipes, tips, and inspiration.

Be Flexible

- **Adapt to Situations**: Be flexible and adapt to different situations, such as eating out or attending social events. Research restaurant menus in advance or bring a plant-based dish to share.
- **Allow Treats**: It's okay to indulge occasionally. Allowing yourself

occasional treats can help prevent feelings of deprivation and make the lifestyle more sustainable.

Monitor Your Health

- **Regular Checkups**: Regularly monitor your health and check in with a healthcare provider. Ensure you are meeting your nutritional needs and make adjustments as necessary.
- **Track Progress**: Keep a journal of your meals, energy levels, and any health changes. Tracking your progress can help you stay motivated and make necessary adjustments.

Celebrate Your Success

- **Acknowledge Achievements**: Celebrate milestones and achievements in your plant-based journey. Recognizing your progress can help keep you motivated.
- **Reward Yourself**: Reward yourself with non-food items or activities that

you enjoy, such as a new book, a day trip, or a spa day.

Transitioning to a whole food plant-based lifestyle can be a rewarding and transformative experience. By following a step-by-step guide, planning your meals, shopping smartly, and making sustainable changes, you can successfully adopt and maintain this healthy lifestyle. In the next chapter, we will provide specific guidance for women over 40, addressing unique health challenges and offering tailored advice for weight loss and chronic disease management.

Chapter 6: Specific Guidance for Women Over 40

Unique Health Challenges

As women age, they encounter unique health challenges that require special attention and care. Understanding these challenges can help women over 40 take proactive steps to maintain and improve their health. Here are some common health issues faced by women in this age group:

Hormonal Changes

- **Menopause**: Around the age of 50, many women experience menopause, which is the cessation of menstrual cycles. This transition can bring about various symptoms such as hot flashes, night sweats, mood swings, and sleep disturbances.
- **Perimenopause**: The period leading up to menopause, known as

perimenopause, can start several years earlier and is characterized by fluctuating hormone levels, irregular periods, and similar symptoms to menopause.

Bone Health

- **Osteoporosis**: As women age, their risk of osteoporosis increases. This condition, characterized by weak and brittle bones, is more common in women due to lower bone density and the decrease in estrogen levels during menopause.

Heart Health

- **Cardiovascular Disease**: Heart disease is the leading cause of death for women. After menopause, the risk of cardiovascular disease increases due to changes in hormone levels, which can affect cholesterol levels and blood vessel health.

Weight Management

- **Metabolic Changes**: Metabolism tends to slow down with age, making it easier to gain weight and harder to lose it. This can lead to increased fat accumulation, particularly around the abdomen.

Mental Health

- **Mental Well-being**: Hormonal fluctuations, life transitions, and the onset of age-related health issues can contribute to anxiety, depression, and other mental health challenges.

Tailored Nutrition Advice

To address these unique health challenges, women over 40 need to focus on specific nutritional needs. A plant-based diet can provide essential nutrients and help manage these issues effectively.

Calcium and Vitamin D

- **Bone Health**: Ensure adequate intake of calcium and vitamin D to support bone health. Good sources of calcium include leafy greens, fortified plant milks, almonds, and tofu. Vitamin D can be obtained from sun exposure, fortified foods, and supplements if necessary.

Phytoestrogens

- **Hormonal Balance**: Phytoestrogens are plant compounds that can mimic the effects of estrogen in the body and help balance hormones. Foods rich in phytoestrogens include flaxseeds, soy products (tofu, tempeh, edamame), and legumes.

Antioxidants

- **Cellular Protection**: Antioxidants help protect cells from damage caused by free radicals. Include a variety of colorful fruits and vegetables in your diet to ensure a good intake of antioxidants. Berries, citrus fruits, leafy greens, and cruciferous vegetables are excellent choices.

Omega-3 Fatty Acids

- **Heart Health**: Omega-3 fatty acids support heart health and reduce inflammation. Plant-based sources of omega-3s include flaxseeds, chia seeds, walnuts, and hemp seeds. Consider an algal oil supplement for DHA and EPA, the active forms of omega-3s.

Fiber

- **Digestive Health and Weight Management**: A high-fiber diet promotes healthy digestion and helps maintain a healthy weight. Incorporate whole grains, fruits, vegetables, legumes, nuts, and seeds into your meals.

B Vitamins

- **Energy and Mental Health**: B vitamins, particularly B12, are essential for energy production and mental health. Fortified foods and supplements are important for ensuring adequate B12 intake on a plant-based diet.

Weight Management

Maintaining a healthy weight becomes more challenging as metabolism slows down with age. However, a plant-based diet can support weight management through nutrient-dense foods that promote satiety and metabolic health.

Eat Nutrient-Dense Foods

- **Whole Foods**: Focus on whole, unprocessed foods that are rich in nutrients and low in empty calories. These foods provide essential vitamins, minerals, and fiber while helping you feel full.

Portion Control

- **Mindful Eating**: Pay attention to portion sizes and practice mindful eating. Listen to your body's hunger and fullness cues, and avoid eating out of boredom or stress.

Regular Physical Activity

- **Stay Active**: Incorporate regular physical activity into your routine to boost metabolism, maintain muscle mass, and promote overall health. Aim for a combination of aerobic exercises, strength training, and flexibility exercises.

Hydration

- **Drink Water**: Staying hydrated is crucial for weight management and overall health. Drink plenty of water throughout the day to support metabolism and prevent overeating.

Balanced Meals

- **Combine Macronutrients**: Create balanced meals that include a mix of protein, healthy fats, and complex carbohydrates. This combination helps stabilize blood sugar levels and keeps you satisfied for longer.

Avoid Processed Foods

- **Minimize Junk Food**: Limit the intake of processed foods, sugary snacks, and high-calorie beverages. These foods can contribute to weight gain and do not provide essential nutrients.

Preventing and Reversing Chronic Diseases

A plant-based diet is highly effective in preventing and reversing many chronic diseases, which become more prevalent with age. Here's how plant-based eating can help:

Heart Disease

- **Lower Cholesterol**: Plant-based diets are naturally low in cholesterol and saturated fats, which can help lower LDL cholesterol levels and reduce the risk of heart disease.
- **Blood Pressure**: High-fiber foods and plant-based nutrients help maintain healthy blood pressure levels.

Diabetes

- **Blood Sugar Control**: Plant-based diets, especially those high in fiber and low in refined sugars, help regulate blood sugar levels and improve insulin sensitivity, reducing the risk of type 2 diabetes.

Cancer

- **Antioxidants and Phytochemicals**: Plant foods are rich in antioxidants and phytochemicals that protect against cancer. Cruciferous

vegetables, berries, and leafy greens
are particularly beneficial.

- **Anti-Inflammatory**: A diet rich in
  anti-inflammatory foods like fruits,
  vegetables, and whole grains can
  reduce the risk of cancer.

Osteoporosis

- **Bone Health**: Adequate calcium and
  vitamin D intake, along with
  weight-bearing exercises, support
  bone health and reduce the risk of
  osteoporosis.

Mental Health

- **Mood and Cognition**: Nutrient-dense
  plant foods provide essential vitamins
  and minerals that support brain health
  and cognitive function. Omega-3 fatty
  acids and B vitamins are particularly
  important for mental well-being.

Digestive Health

- **Healthy Gut**: A high-fiber diet promotes a healthy gut microbiome, improving digestion and reducing the risk of gastrointestinal diseases.

Women over 40 face unique health challenges, but a whole food plant-based diet can provide the necessary nutrients to address these issues effectively. By focusing on nutrient-dense foods, maintaining a healthy weight, and preventing chronic diseases, women can improve their overall health and well-being. The next chapters will provide specific plant-based recipes for breakfast, lunch, dinner, snacks, salads, and drinks to help you implement these dietary changes in a delicious and enjoyable way.

Chapter 7: Plant-Based Breakfast

Starting your day with a nutritious and delicious plant-based breakfast can set the tone for a healthy day. Here are some wholesome breakfast recipes that are easy to prepare, satisfying, and packed with nutrients.

1. Overnight Oats with Berries and Almonds

Ingredients:

- 1 cup rolled oats
- 1 cup almond milk (or any plant milk)
- 1 tablespoon chia seeds
- 1 tablespoon maple syrup (optional)
- 1/2 teaspoon vanilla extract
- 1/2 cup mixed berries (strawberries, blueberries, raspberries)
- 1/4 cup sliced almonds
- 1 tablespoon flaxseed meal (optional)

Directions:

1. In a bowl or jar, combine the rolled oats, almond milk, chia seeds, maple syrup, and vanilla extract. Stir well to combine.
2. Cover and refrigerate overnight, or for at least 4 hours.
3. In the morning, stir the oats. If they are too thick, add a splash of almond milk to reach your desired consistency.
4. Top with mixed berries, sliced almonds, and flaxseed meal if using.
5. Enjoy cold or warm up in the microwave for 1-2 minutes.

Prep Time: 10 minutes
Cook Time: 0 minutes
Servings: 2

2. Tofu Scramble with Spinach and Tomatoes

Ingredients:

- 1 block (14 oz) firm tofu, drained and crumbled
- 1 tablespoon olive oil
- 1 small onion, finely chopped
- 1 garlic clove, minced
- 1 cup cherry tomatoes, halved
- 2 cups fresh spinach leaves
- 1/2 teaspoon turmeric powder
- 1/2 teaspoon cumin powder
- Salt and pepper to taste
- Fresh parsley, chopped (optional)

Directions:

1. Heat the olive oil in a large skillet over medium heat.
2. Add the onion and garlic, and sauté until translucent, about 5 minutes.
3. Add the crumbled tofu, turmeric, and cumin. Stir to combine and cook for another 5 minutes.

4. Add the cherry tomatoes and spinach.
   Cook until the spinach is wilted and
   the tomatoes are soft, about 3-4
   minutes.
5. Season with salt and pepper to taste.
6. Garnish with fresh parsley if desired
   and serve warm.

Prep Time: 10 minutes
Cook Time: 15 minutes
Servings: 2

3. Avocado Toast with Chickpeas and Tahini

Ingredients:

- 2 slices whole grain bread, toasted
- 1 ripe avocado
- 1/2 cup canned chickpeas, drained
  and rinsed
- 1 tablespoon tahini
- 1 tablespoon lemon juice
- Salt and pepper to taste
- Red pepper flakes (optional)

Directions:

1. In a small bowl, mash the avocado with a fork until smooth. Season with salt and pepper.
2. In another bowl, mix the chickpeas with tahini and lemon juice. Use a fork to slightly mash the chickpeas, leaving some whole for texture.
3. Spread the mashed avocado evenly on the toasted bread.
4. Top with the chickpea mixture.
5. Sprinkle with red pepper flakes if desired and serve immediately.

Prep Time: 10 minutes
Cook Time: 0 minutes
Servings: 2

4. Smoothie Bowl with Banana and Spinach

Ingredients:

- 1 banana, frozen and sliced
- 1/2 cup fresh spinach leaves

- 1/2 cup almond milk (or any plant milk)
- 1 tablespoon almond butter
- 1 tablespoon chia seeds
- 1/2 cup granola
- Fresh fruit (berries, kiwi, mango), sliced

Directions:

1. In a blender, combine the frozen banana, spinach, almond milk, almond butter, and chia seeds. Blend until smooth and creamy.
2. Pour the smoothie into a bowl.
3. Top with granola and sliced fresh fruit.
4. Serve immediately with a spoon.

Prep Time: 10 minutes
Cook Time: 0 minutes
Servings: 1

5. Vegan Banana Pancakes

Ingredients:

- 1 cup whole wheat flour
- 1 tablespoon baking powder
- 1 tablespoon sugar (optional)
- 1/2 teaspoon salt
- 1 cup almond milk (or any plant milk)
- 1 ripe banana, mashed
- 1 teaspoon vanilla extract
- 1 tablespoon vegetable oil
- Maple syrup and fresh fruit for serving

Directions:

1. In a large bowl, whisk together the flour, baking powder, sugar (if using), and salt.
2. In another bowl, mix the almond milk, mashed banana, vanilla extract, and vegetable oil until well combined.
3. Pour the wet ingredients into the dry ingredients and stir until just combined. Do not overmix.

4. Heat a non-stick skillet over medium heat and lightly grease with oil.
5. Pour 1/4 cup of batter onto the skillet for each pancake. Cook until bubbles form on the surface, then flip and cook until golden brown, about 2-3 minutes per side.
6. Serve with maple syrup and fresh fruit.

Prep Time: 10 minutes
Cook Time: 15 minutes
Servings: 2

A nutritious and delicious plant-based breakfast is a fantastic way to start your day. These recipes are easy to prepare, packed with nutrients, and will keep you full and energized throughout the morning. Enjoy experimenting with these recipes and feel free to adjust them to your taste preferences. In the next chapter, we will explore plant-based lunch options that are both healthy and satisfying.

Chapter 8: Plant-Based Lunch

A healthy and satisfying plant-based lunch can keep you energized throughout the afternoon and help you maintain focus and productivity. Here are some delicious lunch options that are easy to prepare and packed with nutrients.

1. Quinoa and Black Bean Salad

Ingredients:

- 1 cup quinoa, rinsed
- 2 cups water
- 1 can (15 oz) black beans, drained and rinsed
- 1 cup cherry tomatoes, halved
- 1 cup corn kernels (fresh or frozen)
- 1 red bell pepper, diced
- 1/4 cup red onion, finely chopped
- 1/4 cup fresh cilantro, chopped
- 1 avocado, diced
- Juice of 2 limes

- 2 tablespoons olive oil
- Salt and pepper to taste

Directions:

1. In a medium saucepan, bring the water to a boil. Add the quinoa, reduce the heat to low, cover, and simmer for 15 minutes, or until the quinoa is cooked and water is absorbed. Fluff with a fork and let cool.
2. In a large bowl, combine the cooled quinoa, black beans, cherry tomatoes, corn, red bell pepper, red onion, and cilantro.
3. In a small bowl, whisk together the lime juice, olive oil, salt, and pepper.
4. Pour the dressing over the salad and toss to combine.
5. Gently fold in the diced avocado.
6. Serve immediately or refrigerate until ready to eat.

Prep Time: 15 minutes
Cook Time: 15 minutes
Servings: 4

2. Lentil Soup with Spinach

Ingredients:

- 1 tablespoon olive oil
- 1 onion, finely chopped
- 2 garlic cloves, minced
- 2 carrots, diced
- 2 celery stalks, diced
- 1 cup dried lentils, rinsed
- 1 can (14.5 oz) diced tomatoes
- 6 cups vegetable broth
- 1 teaspoon ground cumin
- 1 teaspoon paprika
- 1/2 teaspoon dried thyme
- Salt and pepper to taste
- 4 cups fresh spinach
- Juice of 1 lemon
- Fresh parsley, chopped (optional)

Directions:

1. Heat the olive oil in a large pot over medium heat.
2. Add the onion, garlic, carrots, and celery. Sauté until the vegetables are softened, about 8 minutes.
3. Stir in the lentils, diced tomatoes, vegetable broth, cumin, paprika, thyme, salt, and pepper.
4. Bring to a boil, then reduce the heat and simmer for 25-30 minutes, or until the lentils are tender.
5. Add the spinach and cook until wilted, about 2 minutes.
6. Stir in the lemon juice and adjust seasoning if needed.
7. Serve hot, garnished with fresh parsley if desired.

Prep Time: 15 minutes
Cook Time: 30 minutes
Servings: 4

3. Chickpea and Avocado Wraps

Ingredients:

- 1 can (15 oz) chickpeas, drained and rinsed
- 1 ripe avocado
- 1 tablespoon lemon juice
- 1 tablespoon tahini
- Salt and pepper to taste
- 1 cup shredded lettuce
- 1/2 cup shredded carrots
- 1/2 cup sliced cucumber
- 4 whole grain wraps

Directions:

1. In a medium bowl, mash the chickpeas and avocado together until mostly smooth.
2. Stir in the lemon juice, tahini, salt, and pepper.
3. Lay out the wraps and divide the chickpea-avocado mixture evenly among them.

4. Top with shredded lettuce, carrots, and cucumber slices.
5. Roll up the wraps tightly and cut in half if desired.
6. Serve immediately or wrap in foil and refrigerate for up to 24 hours.

Prep Time: 10 minutes
Cook Time: 0 minutes
Servings: 4

4. Vegan Buddha Bowl

Ingredients:

- 1 cup brown rice
- 2 cups water
- 1 sweet potato, peeled and diced
- 1 tablespoon olive oil
- Salt and pepper to taste
- 1 can (15 oz) chickpeas, drained and rinsed
- 1 cup steamed broccoli florets
- 1/2 cup shredded red cabbage
- 1/4 cup shredded carrots
- 1/4 cup hummus

- 2 tablespoons tahini
- 2 tablespoons lemon juice
- 1 tablespoon water
- 1 teaspoon maple syrup
- 1/4 teaspoon smoked paprika

Directions:

1. In a medium saucepan, bring the water to a boil. Add the brown rice, reduce the heat, cover, and simmer for 45 minutes or until the rice is cooked and the water is absorbed. Fluff with a fork.
2. Preheat the oven to 400°F (200°C).
3. Toss the diced sweet potato with olive oil, salt, and pepper. Spread on a baking sheet and roast for 25-30 minutes, until tender and lightly browned.
4. In a small bowl, whisk together the tahini, lemon juice, water, maple syrup, and smoked paprika.
5. To assemble the bowls, divide the brown rice among four bowls.

6. Top with roasted sweet potato, chickpeas, steamed broccoli, shredded red cabbage, shredded carrots, and a dollop of hummus.
7. Drizzle with the tahini dressing and serve immediately.

Prep Time: 15 minutes
Cook Time: 45 minutes
Servings: 4

5. Roasted Vegetable and Hummus Sandwich

Ingredients:

- 1 zucchini, sliced
- 1 red bell pepper, sliced
- 1 eggplant, sliced
- 1 tablespoon olive oil
- Salt and pepper to taste
- 1 cup hummus
- 8 slices whole grain bread
- 1 cup fresh spinach leaves

Directions:

1. Preheat the oven to 400°F (200°C).
2. Toss the zucchini, bell pepper, and eggplant slices with olive oil, salt, and pepper.
3. Spread the vegetables on a baking sheet and roast for 20-25 minutes, until tender and slightly charred.
4. Spread a generous layer of hummus on each slice of bread.
5. Layer the roasted vegetables and fresh spinach leaves on four slices of bread, then top with the remaining slices to make sandwiches.
6. Serve immediately or wrap in foil and refrigerate for up to 24 hours.

Prep Time: 10 minutes
Cook Time: 25 minutes
Servings: 4

These plant-based lunch recipes are not only healthy and satisfying but also easy to prepare. They offer a variety of flavors and textures to keep your meals interesting and nutritious. Enjoy these delicious lunch options as part of your plant-based lifestyle, and feel free to customize them to suit your taste preferences. In the next chapter, we will explore plant-based dinner recipes that are hearty and flavorful, perfect for ending your day on a healthy note.

Chapter 9: Plant-Based Dinner

A hearty and flavorful plant-based dinner can be the perfect way to end your day. These recipes are designed to be satisfying, nutritious, and full of flavor. Here are some delicious plant-based dinner options that are easy to prepare and sure to please.

1. Spaghetti with Lentil Bolognese

Ingredients:

- 1 tablespoon olive oil
- 1 onion, finely chopped
- 2 garlic cloves, minced
- 1 carrot, diced
- 1 celery stalk, diced
- 1 cup dried brown or green lentils, rinsed
- 1 can (28 oz) crushed tomatoes
- 3 cups vegetable broth
- 1 teaspoon dried oregano
- 1 teaspoon dried basil

- Salt and pepper to taste
- 12 oz whole grain spaghetti
- Fresh basil, chopped (optional)

Directions:

1. Heat the olive oil in a large pot over medium heat.
2. Add the onion, garlic, carrot, and celery. Sauté until the vegetables are softened, about 8 minutes.
3. Add the lentils, crushed tomatoes, vegetable broth, oregano, basil, salt, and pepper. Bring to a boil, then reduce the heat and simmer for 30-35 minutes, until the lentils are tender.
4. Meanwhile, cook the spaghetti according to the package instructions. Drain and set aside.
5. Serve the lentil Bolognese sauce over the spaghetti and garnish with fresh basil if desired.

Prep Time: 10 minutes
Cook Time: 35 minutes
Servings: 4

2. Chickpea and Vegetable Stir-Fry

Ingredients:

- 1 tablespoon sesame oil
- 1 onion, sliced
- 2 garlic cloves, minced
- 1 red bell pepper, sliced
- 1 yellow bell pepper, sliced
- 1 zucchini, sliced
- 1 cup broccoli florets
- 1 can (15 oz) chickpeas, drained and rinsed
- 3 tablespoons soy sauce or tamari
- 1 tablespoon maple syrup
- 1 tablespoon rice vinegar
- 1 teaspoon grated ginger
- 1 teaspoon cornstarch mixed with 2 tablespoons water
- Cooked brown rice for serving
- Sesame seeds for garnish (optional)

Directions:

1. Heat the sesame oil in a large skillet or wok over medium-high heat.

2. Add the onion and garlic, and sauté for 2-3 minutes until fragrant.
3. Add the bell peppers, zucchini, and broccoli. Stir-fry for 5-7 minutes until the vegetables are tender-crisp.
4. Add the chickpeas and cook for another 2 minutes.
5. In a small bowl, whisk together the soy sauce, maple syrup, rice vinegar, ginger, and cornstarch mixture.
6. Pour the sauce over the vegetables and chickpeas, stirring to coat. Cook for another 2-3 minutes until the sauce thickens.
7. Serve over cooked brown rice and garnish with sesame seeds if desired.

Prep Time: 10 minutes
Cook Time: 15 minutes
Servings: 4

3. Sweet Potato and Black Bean Enchiladas

Ingredients:

- 2 large sweet potatoes, peeled and diced
- 1 tablespoon olive oil
- 1 onion, finely chopped
- 2 garlic cloves, minced
- 1 can (15 oz) black beans, drained and rinsed
- 1 teaspoon ground cumin
- 1 teaspoon chili powder
- Salt and pepper to taste
- 8 whole wheat tortillas
- 2 cups enchilada sauce
- 1/2 cup shredded vegan cheese (optional)
- Fresh cilantro, chopped (optional)

Directions:

1. Preheat the oven to 375°F (190°C).
2. Place the sweet potatoes in a large pot of boiling water. Cook for 10-15

minutes, until tender. Drain and set aside.

3. Heat the olive oil in a large skillet over medium heat. Add the onion and garlic, and sauté until softened, about 5 minutes.

4. Add the black beans, cooked sweet potatoes, cumin, chili powder, salt, and pepper. Stir to combine and cook for another 2-3 minutes.

5. Spread 1/2 cup of enchilada sauce on the bottom of a baking dish.

6. Fill each tortilla with the sweet potato and black bean mixture. Roll up and place seam-side down in the baking dish.

7. Pour the remaining enchilada sauce over the top and sprinkle with vegan cheese if using.

8. Cover with foil and bake for 20 minutes. Remove the foil and bake for an additional 10 minutes.

9. Garnish with fresh cilantro if desired and serve warm.

Prep Time: 15 minutes
Cook Time: 35 minutes
Servings: 4

4. Mushroom and Spinach Risotto

Ingredients:

- 1 tablespoon olive oil
- 1 onion, finely chopped
- 2 garlic cloves, minced
- 2 cups Arborio rice
- 1/2 cup white wine (optional)
- 6 cups vegetable broth, warmed
- 2 cups mushrooms, sliced
- 2 cups fresh spinach leaves
- 1/4 cup nutritional yeast
- Salt and pepper to taste
- Fresh parsley, chopped (optional)

Directions:

1. Heat the olive oil in a large pot over medium heat.
2. Add the onion and garlic, and sauté until softened, about 5 minutes.

3. Add the Arborio rice and cook for 2-3 minutes, stirring frequently, until the rice is slightly translucent.
4. Pour in the white wine, if using, and cook until it has evaporated.
5. Add the vegetable broth one cup at a time, stirring frequently and allowing the liquid to be absorbed before adding more. Continue until the rice is creamy and cooked through, about 18-20 minutes.
6. In a separate skillet, sauté the mushrooms until browned and tender, about 5 minutes.
7. Stir the mushrooms and fresh spinach into the risotto until the spinach is wilted.
8. Stir in the nutritional yeast and season with salt and pepper.
9. Serve warm, garnished with fresh parsley if desired.

Prep Time: 10 minutes
Cook Time: 30 minutes
Servings: 4

5. Thai Red Curry with Vegetables

Ingredients:

- 1 tablespoon coconut oil
- 1 onion, chopped
- 2 garlic cloves, minced
- 1 tablespoon grated ginger
- 2 tablespoons red curry paste
- 1 can (14 oz) coconut milk
- 1 cup vegetable broth
- 1 red bell pepper, sliced
- 1 yellow bell pepper, sliced
- 1 zucchini, sliced
- 1 cup broccoli florets
- 1 cup snap peas
- 1 tablespoon soy sauce or tamari
- 1 teaspoon maple syrup
- Juice of 1 lime
- Fresh basil or cilantro, chopped (optional)
- Cooked jasmine rice for serving

Directions:

1. Heat the coconut oil in a large pot over medium heat.
2. Add the onion, garlic, and ginger. Sauté until fragrant, about 5 minutes.
3. Stir in the red curry paste and cook for another 2 minutes.
4. Pour in the coconut milk and vegetable broth, stirring to combine.
5. Add the red and yellow bell peppers, zucchini, broccoli, and snap peas. Bring to a simmer and cook until the vegetables are tender, about 10-12 minutes.
6. Stir in the soy sauce, maple syrup, and lime juice.
7. Serve over cooked jasmine rice and garnish with fresh basil or cilantro if desired.

Prep Time: 10 minutes
Cook Time: 20 minutes
Servings: 4

These plant-based dinner recipes are hearty, flavorful, and nutritious, providing a satisfying end to your day. By incorporating a variety of vegetables, grains, legumes, and spices, you can create meals that are both delicious and health-promoting. Enjoy experimenting with these recipes and feel free to adjust them to suit your taste preferences. In the next chapter, we will explore plant-based snacks that are tasty and nutritious, perfect for keeping you energized between meals.

Chapter 10: Plant-Based Snacks

Snacking is an important part of a balanced diet, especially when the snacks are nutritious and satisfying. Plant-based snacks can provide the energy and nutrients you need to stay focused and energized throughout the day. Here are some tasty and nutritious snack ideas that are easy to prepare.

1. Energy Balls

Ingredients:

- 1 cup rolled oats
- 1/2 cup almond butter or peanut butter
- 1/4 cup maple syrup or agave nectar
- 1/4 cup chia seeds or flaxseeds
- 1/4 cup dark chocolate chips or raisins
- 1 teaspoon vanilla extract
- Pinch of salt

Directions:

1. In a large bowl, combine all the ingredients and mix well until fully combined.
2. Using your hands, roll the mixture into small balls, about 1 inch in diameter.
3. Place the energy balls on a baking sheet lined with parchment paper.
4. Refrigerate for at least 30 minutes to firm up.
5. Store in an airtight container in the refrigerator for up to a week.

Prep Time: 10 minutes
Cook Time: 0 minutes
Servings: 20 energy balls

2. Hummus and Veggie Sticks

Ingredients:

- 1 can (15 oz) chickpeas, drained and rinsed
- 1/4 cup tahini
- 2 tablespoons olive oil

- Juice of 1 lemon
- 2 garlic cloves, minced
- Salt and pepper to taste
- 1/4 cup water
- Assorted veggies: carrots, cucumbers, bell peppers, celery

Directions:

1. In a food processor, combine the chickpeas, tahini, olive oil, lemon juice, garlic, salt, and pepper.
2. Blend until smooth, adding water as needed to reach your desired consistency.
3. Cut the assorted veggies into sticks.
4. Serve the hummus with veggie sticks for dipping.

Prep Time: 15 minutes
Cook Time: 0 minutes
Servings: 4

3. Baked Kale Chips

Ingredients:

- 1 bunch kale, washed and dried
- 1 tablespoon olive oil
- 1/2 teaspoon salt
- 1/4 teaspoon paprika (optional)

Directions:

1. Preheat the oven to 350°F (175°C).
2. Remove the kale leaves from the stems and tear into bite-sized pieces.
3. In a large bowl, toss the kale with olive oil, salt, and paprika if using.
4. Spread the kale in a single layer on a baking sheet lined with parchment paper.
5. Bake for 10-15 minutes, until the edges are crispy but not burnt.
6. Allow to cool before serving.

Prep Time: 10 minutes
Cook Time: 15 minutes
Servings: 4

4. Almond and Date Bars

Ingredients:

- 1 cup almonds
- 1 cup pitted dates
- 1/4 cup shredded coconut
- 1 tablespoon coconut oil
- 1 teaspoon vanilla extract
- Pinch of salt

Directions:

1. In a food processor, pulse the almonds until finely chopped.
2. Add the dates, shredded coconut, coconut oil, vanilla extract, and salt. Process until the mixture comes together and forms a sticky dough.
3. Press the mixture into an 8x8-inch baking dish lined with parchment paper.
4. Refrigerate for at least 1 hour to firm up.

5. Cut into bars and store in an airtight container in the refrigerator for up to a week.

Prep Time: 10 minutes
Cook Time: 0 minutes (plus 1 hour chilling time)
Servings: 12 bars

5. Chia Pudding

Ingredients:

- 1/4 cup chia seeds
- 1 cup almond milk (or any plant milk)
- 1 tablespoon maple syrup or agave nectar
- 1/2 teaspoon vanilla extract
- Fresh fruit for topping (e.g., berries, mango, banana)

Directions:

1. In a bowl, combine the chia seeds, almond milk, maple syrup, and vanilla extract. Stir well to combine.

2. Cover and refrigerate for at least 2
   hours, or overnight, until the chia
   seeds have absorbed the liquid and the
   mixture has thickened.
3. Stir the pudding again before serving.
4. Top with fresh fruit and enjoy.

Prep Time: 5 minutes
Cook Time: 0 minutes (plus 2 hours chilling time)
Servings: 2

6. Roasted Chickpeas

Ingredients:

- 1 can (15 oz) chickpeas, drained and rinsed
- 1 tablespoon olive oil
- 1 teaspoon paprika
- 1/2 teaspoon garlic powder
- 1/2 teaspoon salt
- 1/4 teaspoon black pepper

Directions:

1. Preheat the oven to 400°F (200°C).

2. Pat the chickpeas dry with a paper towel.
3. In a bowl, toss the chickpeas with olive oil, paprika, garlic powder, salt, and pepper.
4. Spread the chickpeas in a single layer on a baking sheet lined with parchment paper.
5. Roast for 20-30 minutes, shaking the pan halfway through, until the chickpeas are crispy.
6. Allow to cool before serving.

Prep Time: 10 minutes
Cook Time: 20-30 minutes
Servings: 4

7. Fruit and Nut Mix

Ingredients:

- 1/2 cup almonds
- 1/2 cup walnuts
- 1/2 cup cashews
- 1/2 cup dried cranberries
- 1/2 cup raisins

- 1/2 cup dark chocolate chips
  (optional)

Directions:

1. In a large bowl, combine all the
   ingredients and mix well.
2. Store in an airtight container.

Prep Time: 5 minutes
Cook Time: 0 minutes
Servings: 8

8. Apple Slices with Almond Butter

Ingredients:

- 2 apples, cored and sliced
- 1/4 cup almond butter
- 1 tablespoon chia seeds or flaxseeds
  (optional)

Directions:

1. Arrange the apple slices on a plate.
2. Serve with almond butter for dipping.
3. Sprinkle chia seeds or flaxseeds on
   top of the almond butter if desired.

Prep Time: 5 minutes
Cook Time: 0 minutes
Servings: 2

These plant-based snacks are not only delicious and satisfying but also packed with nutrients that will keep you energized throughout the day. Enjoy experimenting with these recipes and feel free to adjust them to suit your taste preferences. In the next chapter, we will explore plant-based salads that are creative, filling, and perfect for any meal.

Chapter 11: Plant-Based Salads

Salads can be a nutritious and satisfying part of any meal. They are versatile, easy to prepare, and can be packed with a variety of textures and flavors. Here are some creative and filling plant-based salad recipes that are perfect for any occasion.

1. Mediterranean Quinoa Salad

Ingredients:

- 1 cup quinoa, rinsed
- 2 cups water
- 1 cup cherry tomatoes, halved
- 1 cucumber, diced
- 1 red bell pepper, diced
- 1/4 cup red onion, finely chopped
- 1/4 cup Kalamata olives, pitted and sliced
- 1/4 cup fresh parsley, chopped
- 1/4 cup fresh mint, chopped
- 1/4 cup lemon juice

- 3 tablespoons olive oil
- Salt and pepper to taste

Directions:

1. In a medium saucepan, bring the water to a boil. Add the quinoa, reduce the heat to low, cover, and simmer for 15 minutes, or until the quinoa is cooked and the water is absorbed. Fluff with a fork and let cool.
2. In a large bowl, combine the cooked quinoa, cherry tomatoes, cucumber, red bell pepper, red onion, olives, parsley, and mint.
3. In a small bowl, whisk together the lemon juice, olive oil, salt, and pepper.
4. Pour the dressing over the salad and toss to combine.
5. Serve immediately or refrigerate until ready to eat.

Prep Time: 15 minutes
Cook Time: 15 minutes
Servings: 4

2. Sweet Potato and Black Bean Salad

Ingredients:

- 2 large sweet potatoes, peeled and diced
- 1 tablespoon olive oil
- 1 teaspoon cumin
- 1 teaspoon paprika
- Salt and pepper to taste
- 1 can (15 oz) black beans, drained and rinsed
- 1 red bell pepper, diced
- 1 avocado, diced
- 1/4 cup red onion, finely chopped
- 1/4 cup fresh cilantro, chopped
- 1 lime, juiced
- 2 tablespoons olive oil
- 1 teaspoon maple syrup

Directions:

1. Preheat the oven to 400°F (200°C).
2. Toss the diced sweet potatoes with olive oil, cumin, paprika, salt, and pepper. Spread on a baking sheet and roast for 25-30 minutes, until tender and lightly browned. Let cool.
3. In a large bowl, combine the roasted sweet potatoes, black beans, red bell pepper, avocado, red onion, and cilantro.
4. In a small bowl, whisk together the lime juice, olive oil, and maple syrup.
5. Pour the dressing over the salad and toss to combine.
6. Serve immediately or refrigerate until ready to eat.

Prep Time: 15 minutes
Cook Time: 30 minutes
Servings: 4

3. Asian Edamame Salad

Ingredients:

- 2 cups shelled edamame (fresh or frozen)
- 1 cup shredded red cabbage
- 1 cup shredded carrots
- 1 red bell pepper, thinly sliced
- 3 green onions, chopped
- 1/4 cup fresh cilantro, chopped
- 1/4 cup roasted peanuts, chopped
- 3 tablespoons soy sauce or tamari
- 2 tablespoons rice vinegar
- 1 tablespoon sesame oil
- 1 tablespoon maple syrup
- 1 teaspoon grated ginger
- 1 teaspoon sesame seeds (optional)

Directions:

1. If using frozen edamame, cook according to package instructions and let cool.
2. In a large bowl, combine the edamame, red cabbage, carrots, red

bell pepper, green onions, cilantro, and peanuts.
3. In a small bowl, whisk together the soy sauce, rice vinegar, sesame oil, maple syrup, and grated ginger.
4. Pour the dressing over the salad and toss to combine.
5. Sprinkle with sesame seeds if desired and serve.

Prep Time: 15 minutes
Cook Time: 5 minutes (if cooking edamame)
Servings: 4

4. Lentil and Roasted Beet Salad

Ingredients:

- 1 cup lentils, rinsed
- 2 cups water
- 3 medium beets, peeled and diced
- 1 tablespoon olive oil
- Salt and pepper to taste
- 2 cups arugula
- 1/4 cup walnuts, toasted and chopped

- 1/4 cup vegan feta cheese (optional)
- 3 tablespoons balsamic vinegar
- 2 tablespoons olive oil
- 1 tablespoon Dijon mustard
- 1 teaspoon maple syrup

Directions:

1. Preheat the oven to 400°F (200°C).
2. Toss the diced beets with olive oil, salt, and pepper. Spread on a baking sheet and roast for 30-35 minutes, until tender and lightly browned. Let cool.
3. In a medium saucepan, bring the water to a boil. Add the lentils, reduce the heat to low, cover, and simmer for 20-25 minutes, or until the lentils are tender. Drain and let cool.
4. In a large bowl, combine the cooked lentils, roasted beets, arugula, walnuts, and vegan feta cheese if using.
5. In a small bowl, whisk together the balsamic vinegar, olive oil, Dijon mustard, and maple syrup.

6. Pour the dressing over the salad and toss to combine.

7. Serve immediately or refrigerate until ready to eat.

Prep Time: 15 minutes
Cook Time: 35 minutes
Servings: 4

5. Mexican Corn and Avocado Salad

Ingredients:

- 4 ears of corn, grilled or boiled, kernels removed
- 1 can (15 oz) black beans, drained and rinsed
- 1 red bell pepper, diced
- 1 avocado, diced
- 1/4 cup red onion, finely chopped
- 1/4 cup fresh cilantro, chopped
- 1 lime, juiced
- 2 tablespoons olive oil
- 1 teaspoon cumin
- Salt and pepper to taste

Directions:

1. In a large bowl, combine the corn kernels, black beans, red bell pepper, avocado, red onion, and cilantro.
2. In a small bowl, whisk together the lime juice, olive oil, cumin, salt, and pepper.
3. Pour the dressing over the salad and toss to combine.
4. Serve immediately or refrigerate until ready to eat.

Prep Time: 15 minutes
Cook Time: 10 minutes (if grilling or boiling corn)
Servings: 4

These plant-based salads are not only creative and filling but also packed with nutrients to keep you energized and satisfied.

Enjoy experimenting with these recipes and feel free to adjust them to suit your taste preferences. In the next chapter, we will explore plant-based drinks that are refreshing and healthful, perfect for any time of day.

Chapter 12: Plant-Based Drinks

Refreshing and healthful beverages can be a wonderful addition to your plant-based lifestyle. These drinks are not only delicious but also packed with nutrients. Here are some delightful recipes for smoothies, juices, and other plant-based beverages.

1. Green Detox Smoothie

Ingredients:

- 1 cup spinach leaves
- 1 banana
- 1 apple, cored and chopped
- 1/2 cucumber, chopped
- 1 tablespoon chia seeds
- 1 cup coconut water
- Juice of 1 lemon

Directions:

1. Combine all ingredients in a blender.
2. Blend until smooth and creamy.
3. Pour into a glass and serve immediately.

Prep Time: 5 minutes
Cook Time: 0 minutes
Servings: 2

2. Berry Banana Smoothie

Ingredients:

- 1 banana
- 1 cup mixed berries (strawberries, blueberries, raspberries)
- 1 cup almond milk (or any plant milk)
- 1 tablespoon flaxseed meal
- 1 teaspoon vanilla extract

Directions:

1. Combine all ingredients in a blender.
2. Blend until smooth and creamy.
3. Pour into a glass and serve immediately.

Prep Time: 5 minutes
Cook Time: 0 minutes
Servings: 2

3. Golden Turmeric Latte

Ingredients:

- 2 cups almond milk (or any plant milk)
- 1 teaspoon ground turmeric
- 1/2 teaspoon ground cinnamon
- 1/4 teaspoon ground ginger
- 1 tablespoon maple syrup (optional)
- Pinch of black pepper

Directions:

1. In a small saucepan, combine the almond milk, turmeric, cinnamon, ginger, maple syrup, and black pepper.
2. Heat over medium heat, whisking continuously, until the mixture is hot but not boiling.
3. Pour into mugs and serve immediately.

Prep Time: 5 minutes
Cook Time: 5 minutes
Servings: 2

4. Refreshing Cucumber Mint Water

Ingredients:

- 1 cucumber, thinly sliced
- 1/4 cup fresh mint leaves
- 1 lemon, thinly sliced
- 8 cups water

Directions:

1. In a large pitcher, combine the cucumber, mint leaves, and lemon slices.
2. Fill the pitcher with water.
3. Refrigerate for at least 1 hour before serving.

Prep Time: 5 minutes
Cook Time: 0 minutes
Servings: 8

5. Vegan Hot Chocolate

Ingredients:

- 2 cups almond milk (or any plant milk)
- 2 tablespoons cocoa powder
- 2 tablespoons maple syrup or agave nectar
- 1/2 teaspoon vanilla extract
- Pinch of salt

Directions:

1. In a small saucepan, combine the almond milk, cocoa powder, maple syrup, vanilla extract, and salt.
2. Heat over medium heat, whisking continuously, until the mixture is hot but not boiling.
3. Pour into mugs and serve immediately.

Prep Time: 5 minutes
Cook Time: 5 minutes
Servings: 2

Bonus: Other Recipes

These additional recipes are perfect for various occasions, from a quick snack to a special treat.

1. Avocado Toast

Ingredients:

- 2 slices whole grain bread, toasted
- 1 ripe avocado
- Salt and pepper to taste
- Red pepper flakes (optional)

Directions:

1. Mash the avocado in a small bowl.
2. Spread the mashed avocado on the toasted bread.
3. Season with salt, pepper, and red pepper flakes if desired.
4. Serve immediately.

Prep Time: 5 minutes
Cook Time: 0 minutes
Servings: 1

2. Vegan Chocolate Mousse

Ingredients:

- 1 can (15 oz) coconut milk, refrigerated overnight
- 1/4 cup cocoa powder
- 1/4 cup maple syrup or agave nectar
- 1 teaspoon vanilla extract

Directions:

1. Scoop the solidified coconut cream from the top of the can into a mixing bowl, discarding the liquid.
2. Add the cocoa powder, maple syrup, and vanilla extract.
3. Whip with an electric mixer until light and fluffy.
4. Spoon into serving dishes and refrigerate for at least 1 hour before serving.

Prep Time: 10 minutes
Cook Time: 0 minutes (plus 1 hour chilling time)
Servings: 4

3. Chickpea Salad Sandwich

Ingredients:

- 1 can (15 oz) chickpeas, drained and rinsed
- 1/4 cup vegan mayonnaise
- 1 tablespoon Dijon mustard
- 1 tablespoon lemon juice
- 1 celery stalk, finely chopped
- 1 green onion, finely chopped
- Salt and pepper to taste
- 4 slices whole grain bread
- Lettuce leaves

Directions:

1. In a bowl, mash the chickpeas with a fork.
2. Stir in the vegan mayonnaise, Dijon mustard, lemon juice, celery, green onion, salt, and pepper.
3. Spread the chickpea salad on two slices of bread.
4. Top with lettuce leaves and the remaining slices of bread.

5. Serve immediately.

Prep Time: 10 minutes
Cook Time: 0 minutes
Servings: 2

4. Mango Coconut Chia Pudding

Ingredients:

- 1/4 cup chia seeds
- 1 cup coconut milk
- 1 tablespoon maple syrup or agave nectar
- 1 ripe mango, diced

Directions:

1. In a bowl, combine the chia seeds, coconut milk, and maple syrup. Stir well.
2. Cover and refrigerate for at least 2 hours, or overnight, until the chia seeds have absorbed the liquid and the mixture has thickened.
3. Stir the pudding again before serving.
4. Top with diced mango and serve.

Prep Time: 5 minutes

Cook Time: 0 minutes (plus 2 hours chilling time)

Servings: 2

5. Spicy Roasted Chickpeas

Ingredients:

- 1 can (15 oz) chickpeas, drained and rinsed
- 1 tablespoon olive oil
- 1 teaspoon paprika
- 1/2 teaspoon cumin
- 1/2 teaspoon garlic powder
- 1/4 teaspoon cayenne pepper (optional)
- Salt and pepper to taste

Directions:

1. Preheat the oven to 400°F (200°C).
2. Pat the chickpeas dry with a paper towel.
3. In a bowl, toss the chickpeas with olive oil, paprika, cumin, garlic

powder, cayenne pepper, salt, and pepper.

4. Spread the chickpeas in a single layer on a baking sheet lined with parchment paper.
5. Roast for 20-30 minutes, shaking the pan halfway through, until the chickpeas are crispy.
6. Allow to cool before serving.

Prep Time: 10 minutes
Cook Time: 20-30 minutes
Servings: 4

These plant-based drinks and additional recipes are refreshing, nutritious, and easy to prepare. Whether you're looking for a quick snack, a satisfying beverage, or a special treat, these recipes offer something for everyone. Enjoy incorporating these delightful options into your plant-based lifestyle, and feel free to experiment with variations to suit your taste preferences.

Conclusion

Key Takeaways

Throughout this book, we have explored the transformative power of a whole food plant-based diet. Here are the key takeaways to remember as you embark on your plant-powered journey:

1. **Health Transformation**: A whole food plant-based diet can prevent, manage, and even reverse chronic diseases such as heart disease, diabetes, and cancer.
2. **Nutritional Essentials**: It's possible to meet all your nutritional needs, including protein, calcium, vitamin B12, vitamin D, and omega-3s, through a well-planned plant-based diet.
3. **Weight Management**: Plant-based eating aids in weight loss and maintenance without feelings of

deprivation by focusing on nutrient-dense, low-calorie foods.

4. **Transitioning**: Transitioning to a plant-based lifestyle can be simple and sustainable with the right steps, meal planning, grocery shopping tips, and understanding your nutritional needs.

5. **Special Considerations**: Women over 40 can particularly benefit from plant-based nutrition, addressing unique health challenges and promoting overall well-being.

6. **Delicious Recipes**: Enjoying a variety of delicious, nutritious meals—from breakfast to dinner, snacks, salads, and drinks—makes the plant-based lifestyle enjoyable and fulfilling.

Encouragement

Embracing a plant-based lifestyle is a powerful step towards better health and a more sustainable world. By making conscious food choices, you are investing in your health, protecting the environment, and contributing to the well-being of all living beings. Remember that every small change you make can have a significant impact. Celebrate your progress, stay informed, and seek support from the plant-based community.

Your journey may have challenges, but with determination and the wealth of resources available, you can overcome them. You have the tools and knowledge to take control of your health destiny. Start today, embrace the plant-powered life, and experience the incredible benefits that come with it.

Acknowledgments

I would like to express my heartfelt gratitude to everyone who has supported me throughout this journey. To my family and friends, thank you for your support and encouragement. To my clients and followers, your dedication to improving your health through plant-based eating inspires me every day.

Special thanks to the Plant-Based Nutrition community and all the researchers, authors, and advocates whose work has been instrumental in advancing the understanding of plant-based health. Your contributions have made this book possible.

Lastly, thank you to my readers. Your interest and commitment to a healthier lifestyle are what drive me to continue this important work. I hope this book has provided you with valuable insights and practical tools to embrace plant-powered life. Together, we can make a positive

impact on our health and the world around
us.

www.ingramcontent.com/pod-product-compliance
Lightning Source LLC
Chambersburg PA
CBHW070840250726
48662CB00003B/1309